Hormones and Diet In Women:

A Game-Plan for Women to Achieve Hormonal Balance and Shed Weight.

By

LENA R JOHNSON

COPYRIGHT

TABLE OF CONTENTS

Hormones & Diet in Women

INTRODUCTION

The majority of diet programs are designed with men in mind, yet women's bodies function differently. Because popular programs can have a detrimental effect on a woman's sensitive and complex hormonal system, they may make it more difficult for women to lose weight. Through tailored treatment, this book, 'Hormones and diet in Women: a game-plan for Women to Achieve Hormonal Balance and shed weight' has helped women understand hormonal difficulties and enhance their overall health. Lena R. Johnson offers a revolutionary game plan in her book that enables women to regulate their hormones and reduce extra weight, improving their health. These has offered a fat-burning method that works, including hormone cleansing, a ketogenic diet designed specifically for women, an intermittent fasting schedule, and satisfying dishes.

In this book, we will explore the language of hormones and how women's food and hormone production are misunderstood.

Hormones & Diet in Women

Sex hormones have been linked to a number of serious clinical diseases in women and are crucial in controlling appetite, eating habits, and energy metabolism.

Progesterone and testosterone may increase hunger, whereas estrogen suppresses the desire to eat. This review outlines new research on the relationship between neuroendocrine processes and sex hormones in the regulation of female hunger and eating behavior. In addition, we are learning more about the roles that sex hormones play in the emergence of obesity and eating problems. For example, androgens may exacerbate bulimia by increasing appetite and decreasing self-control; this theory is corroborated by the finding that antiandrogenic therapy lessens bulimic behavior.

The etiology of female abdominal obesity also involves androgens. On the other hand, the weight increase and buildup of belly fat linked to the menopausal transition are countered by hormone replacement therapy with estrogen. To sum up, sex hormones and/or substances with comparable properties might offer new approaches to treating eating disorders and obesity, two of the biggest health issues facing women nowadays.

Hormones & Diet in Women

In my experience, women come to me frequently, exhausted, irritable, stressed, and always bemoaning the extra weight they gain, even though they try their hardest to exercise and eat healthily. These problems typically arise for women as they approach their mid-30s. Many women have noticed that it's more difficult to maintain a healthy weight; even with January's discipline, those holiday pounds are harder to shed. What's even more discouraging is that diets that used to work for their male coworkers and partners don't seem to work the same for them. When I tell women that the answer to their symptoms lies not in calorie counting or treadmill miles but rather in learning to speak the language of hormones, they are often taken aback. You may be wondering what I mean when I say that hormones are the key to true health science that honors their bodies. Well, as a healthcare provider, I can tell you without a doubt that you cannot achieve true health science that honors your body. What I mean is that when your diet and lifestyle support your hormones, it's like a cool breeze on a hot summer day when your food tells your body to burn fat and promote health.

You flip a metabolic switch, and your body is transformed, especially after age 35, when the body becomes more difficult to move and your metabolism slows down.

CHAPTER 1
Understanding Your Hormones

The human body has more than 200 hormones. The most well-known hormones include thyroid, cortisol, insulin, leptin, ghrelin, and estrogen. These have a tight relationship with mood, fertility, and metabolism. Human growth hormone (HGH), as it is also called somatotropin, is a naturally occurring hormone that your pituitary gland produces and releases. It acts on various parts of the body to support children's growth.

Your body still needs growth hormones even after the growth plates (epiphyses) in your bones have fused. HGH aids in the maintenance of normal body composition and metabolism once growth is complete, which includes regulating blood sugar (glucose) levels to a safe range. A tiny, pea-sized endocrine gland, the pituitary is situated beneath the hypothalamus at the base of the brain. The anterior (front) lobe and the posterior (back) lobe make up this structure.

Hormones & Diet in Women

HGH is produced by your anterior lobe. Your hypothalamus and pituitary gland are linked by a network of nerves and blood vessels. The pituitary stalk is the term for this. The area of the brain that regulates bodily temperature, heart rate, blood pressure, and digestion is called the hypothalamus. Your hypothalamus instructs your pituitary gland to release specific hormones by communicating with it through the stalk.

Growth hormone-releasing hormones (GHRH) are released by the hypothalamus, while somatostatin inhibits (prevents) the production of HGH by the pituitary gland. Healthcare professionals treat several illnesses, such as growth hormone insufficiency, with synthetic human growth hormone (also known as recombinant HGH). Synthetic HGH should never be used without a prescription from a physician.

Chapter 2
The Metabolic Process of hormones

Insulin: After a meal, the pancreas releases insulin, which transports glucose (sugar) from the blood to the cells where it is needed for energy.

Additionally, insulin is the hormone that causes excess sugar to be stored as fat.

Released from fat cells, **leptin** helps regulate hunger, maintain body weight, and alert the brain when a person is full. This hormone is commonly known as the **"satiety hormone."**

Ghrelin: Also referred to as the "hunger hormone," this hormone stimulates your appetite.

Thyroid hormones: thyroxine (T4) and triiodothyronine (T3) control temperature, energy levels, weight, and the growth of hair, skin, and nails, among other things.

The Essential Function Of Hormones In Human Health

To help manage and govern your body's development, hormones are molecules that are produced within and transferred throughout it. Both important life events and many of our everyday activities depend heavily on them. Blood pressure, blood sugar, growth and fertility, sex desire, metabolism, and even sleep are all impacted by hormones. They can have such an impact that they alter our daily thoughts and behaviors. No one can deny the power of hormones.

Why Do Hormones Affect Women Differently Than Men?

Menopause, pregnancy, and adolescence are just a few of the significant life events that are influenced by hormonal shifts in females. Except during puberty, men do not experience high amounts of hormone swings while having the same hormones as women.

Hormones & Diet in Women

Hormonal changes in women tend to be more abrupt and regular. Difficult symptoms may result from these changes for some people.

Hormone Impact On The Body And The Mind

We often attribute hormones to a variety of symptoms and illnesses. When crafting a health narrative or discussing a health ailment, "Whenever I talk to experts on the phone, they always say, 'Hormones, hormones.'" So that's it. We'll just blame hormones for it. Bloating, acne, or sore breasts are possible side effects of ovulation and premenstrual syndrome.

Fatigue and cramps are common during menstruation. Indeed, numerous physical changes come with pregnancy. Night sweats, dry vaginas, and hot flashes can all be symptoms of menopause.

Hormones & Diet in Women

Psychological repercussions also exist. A common complaint among women during these hormonal shifts is mood swings, anxiety, irritability, insomnia, and other behavioral abnormalities. "Mood and anxiety are greatly influenced by hormones." A variety of hormones are the cause. In reality, the hormone estrogen acts as an antidepressant within your brain. Anxiety or depression may result from an overactive or underactive thyroid. The stress hormone cortisol has an impact on mood. Thus, the impacts on the brain are rather significant overall.

When Do Hormones Become Problematic?

"Either elevated or decreased hormone levels can be controlled by the brain and still be okay." i.e., the constant fluctuation of hormones is where problems arise. Some ladies take that more personally than others. Patients frequently only mention that they feel "off" or not themselves when they visit their doctor.

Although hormone levels can be measured through laboratory work, a lot of professionals concurred that whether or not hormone levels are hurting someone's quality of life is more significant.

"Is it getting to the point where you're having significant trouble sleeping or eating?" experts demonstrated how to decide if you should seek assistance. Does it affect your focus, memory, productivity, or ability to complete tasks during the day? Does this have a big impact on your relationships? Does it give you trouble at work?" Here speaking with a medical practitioner should be the first step in discussing any suicidal thoughts or sentiments.

Options for therapy

One of the most widespread misconceptions regarding hormones is that there is nothing we can do to enhance our quality of life or lessen the symptoms.

Hormones & Diet in Women

There are numerous possibilities for treatment. However, the treatment must be customized to the patient's specific condition to be effective. The first thing to do is to locate the source of the disruptions. Though easily treated physical problems may be the primary cause, our mood may be most affected. The psychological effects of these fundamental motor symptoms are making it difficult for many people to respond. You can start down the path to a treatment plan that works for you by talking with your doctor about your concerns. It's a conversation between two people. I don't know you, so I would never just advise, "Take this, take that." "Every woman needs to have this conversation on her own." There are numerous options and combinations for medical care. Hormonal drugs, for instance, come in a wide variety. Furthermore, choosing what you like is not always easy; some trial and error is typically required to discover the best fit. "The important thing is that it's customized."

Hormones & Diet in Women

No one can benefit from the same prescription. You would need to have a serious conversation with someone about your day and nighttime routine and what we can do to support you.

Exercise And Diet

Beyond medicine, a lot of professionals advise eating well and exercising to lessen the negative effects of hormone fluctuations on the body and mind. "Workout comes first. Stress is a major factor in determining any kind of mood or anxiety symptom that results from hormonal changes. Therefore, you perform far better when your stress levels are low. You function far worse when you're under a lot of stress.

I don't care if you go to a gym if you can afford to go to a gym or if you buy $3 ankle weights and walk around the block ten times. Another option is to simply raise your legs against gravity while sitting on a chair. It will also lift your spirits, so you should be doing something for your bones.

Hormones & Diet in Women

Maintaining one's health and emotional state can both benefit from a diet. Consuming a range of fruits and vegetables, lean proteins, and avoiding alcohol can all help with energy levels, improve sleep patterns, help you maintain a healthy weight, and supply the right amounts of vitamins and minerals. A nutritious diet can support the brain's optimal functioning if the brain's reaction to fluctuating hormones plays a significant role in an individual's experience. The building blocks must come from your food. Research has emphasized that nutrients like folate and B12 are quickly absorbed by the brain. " It's important to get as much information as possible into your brain in order to improve its efficiency."

CHAPTER 3
Here Are The Ten(10) Signs Of A Hormone Imbalance

Diverse Emotions Or Mood Swing

The female sex hormone estrogen affects brain neurotransmitters, including the mood-enhancing hormone serotonin. Estrogen variations may be the cause of premenstrual syndrome (PMS) or sadness during perimenopause (the period of time before periods completely stop).

Heaviness of Period Or Unease

You may have fibroids if you also experience other symptoms including lower back pain, constipation, poor erections, abdominal pain, or painful sex. Fibroids are non-cancerous growths in or near the womb. Estrogen is thought to be the trigger, however, the precise cause is unknown; a family history may potentially predispose you.

Low Motivation/low libido

Low libido is especially common in women going through perimenopause or menopause due to falling levels of estrogen and testosterone (yes, testosterone is a hormone found in women, despite being associated with males).

Additional menopausal symptoms including concern, tiredness, low mood, and night sweats may also impact your sexual life.

Insomnia And Poor Quality Of Sleep

During perimenopause and menopause, the ovaries gradually decrease the synthesis of progesterone and estrogen, which promotes sleep. Diminished estrogen levels may also play a role in night sweats, which can disrupt sleep, result in fatigue, and sap vitality.

Gaining Weight Unintentionally

Many hormone-related disorders can lead to weight gain, including underactive thyroid syndrome (where the thyroid gland produces insufficient thyroid hormones to regulate metabolism), menopause (which causes hormonal changes that can increase the likelihood of gaining weight around the abdomen), and PCOS (polycystic ovary syndrome), which is characterized by small ovarian cysts.

Cutaneous/Skin Problems

Persistent adult acne may be a sign of polycystic ovarian syndrome, low progesterone and estrogen levels, and high levels of androgen hormones. Similarly, dry skin can be caused by thyroid problems or the menopause, while itchy skin might be caused by hormone imbalances during pregnancy or the menopause.

Problems During Conception/infertility

One of the main causes of hormonal imbalance in female infertility is changing hormone levels, which cause a woman's fertility to typically diminish after the age of 35. Low levels of luteinizing hormone (LH), which triggers the ovaries to release an egg and start producing progesterone, can also lead to fertility problems. A woman's likelihood of getting pregnant can be decreased by high levels of the hormone follicle-stimulating hormone (FSH). Reproductive problems such as PCOS and early menopause will affect your ability to conceive.

A Migraine/Headache

Many women have headaches due to hormonal imbalances brought on by menstruation, pregnancy, or menopause.

Delicate Bones

Bone loss may occur from decreased estrogen levels throughout the perimenopause and menopause.

Hormones & Diet in Women

Drier Genitalia/Vagina dryness

The main reason of vaginal dryness is a drop in estrogen levels, especially throughout the perimenopause and menopause. Hormone level fluctuations brought on by antidepressant medications or the contraceptive pill might potentially cause the problem.

Hormone Imbalance Symptoms

Because hormones control every aspect of your health, symptoms of a hormone imbalance might manifest in different sections of your body. While not all signs of hormone imbalance are indicative of a problem, some are more likely to indicate that your hormones could use some attention than others.

- Weariness

- Perceptiveness

- Dim desire

Hormones & Diet in Women

- Reluctance to lose weight

- Weight reduction that is rapid

- Hair thinning or loss

- Frequent headaches and migraines

- Problems with blood sugar and cravings

- Dizzy thinking

- Variations in timing

The PMS.

- Pores

- Depressed state

CHAPTER 4
Foods that Balance Hormones

How Maintaining a Healthy Diet Can Help Your Hormones.
Hormone imbalances can lead to a variety of issues, including diabetes and infertility, but some foods can help maintain hormonal balance and optimal bodily function. We discuss the foods that are best for hormone health. Hormones may not always be the first thing that comes to mind when we consider what to eat to fuel our bodies. However, our bodies depend heavily on our hormones. The endocrine system's chemical messengers, or hormones, aid in growth and development, metabolism and digestion, fertility, stress management, mood, and a host of other functions. A hormonal imbalance can result in a variety of disorders, including diabetes, weight gain or loss, and infertility. An imbalance can also be caused by something interfering with signaling pathways or insufficient or excessive production of hormones.

Hormones & Diet in Women

A balanced diet can support hormonal homeostasis. Here's a summary of the things your hormones regulate and the nutrients that help maintain their balance.

Hormone Effects of Diet

Hormone synthesis and its signaling pathways are influenced by our diet. "On the other hand, pesticides, alcohol, and artificial sweeteners can negatively affect hormones. Our protein hormones like healthy fats, olive oil, avocado, nuts, and seeds, as well as ample fiber from fruits and vegetables and quality proteins, like eggs, fish, and meat, also require an adequate amount of calories. Women's bodies are particularly vulnerable to shortages. Your body will lower the amount of sex hormones produced if it feels as though it isn't getting enough. Your body is incapable of distinguishing between a new weight-loss diet that you are trying out and a famine, a war, or both.

How to Detect an Imbalance in Hormones.

"During the reproductive years, women can look to their cycle for clues about the state of their hormones: headaches, heavy painful periods, PMS, and infertility are all examples of "period disorders" that indicate an imbalance in hormones.

Unusual swings in weight or energy levels may also indicate a hormone imbalance. However, the only reliable way to be certain is to test.

CHAPTER 5
All-Natural Strategies for Hormone Balancing

Consume Adequate Protein At Each Meal.

It is crucial to include enough protein in your diet. In addition to providing your body with necessary amino acids that it is unable to create on its own, protein is also necessary for the production of peptide hormones, or hormones produced from proteins. These hormones are produced by your endocrine glands using amino acids. Numerous physiological functions, including development, energy metabolism, appetite, stress, and reproduction, are significantly influenced by peptide hormones.

For instance, eating enough protein affects hormones that regulate hunger and food consumption and alert your brain about your energy level.

Exercise On A Regular Basis

Hormonal health is highly influenced by physical activity. Exercise boosts hormone receptor sensitivity, which means that it improves the transport of nutrients and hormone signals in addition to increasing blood flow to your muscles. Exercise's capacity to lower insulin levels and raise insulin sensitivity is one of its main advantages. A hormone called insulin enables cells to absorb blood sugar and use it as fuel. On the other hand, your cells cannot respond to insulin as well if you have a condition known as insulin resistance. This illness increases the risk of heart disease, diabetes, and obesity.

Continue To Weigh Moderately.

Hormonal abnormalities linked to weight gain can cause issues with insulin sensitivity and reproductive health.

Hormones & Diet in Women

Insulin resistance is closely associated with obesity, and insulin resistance is positively correlated with weight loss, which lowers the risk of diabetes and heart disease as well as improves insulin resistance. Hypogonadism, or decreased or absent hormone release from the ovaries or testes, is also linked to obesity.

In fact, for those who are born with a male sex assignment, this disorder is among the most significant hormonal side effects of obesity. This indicates that in individuals assigned female at birth, obesity relates to a lack of ovulation and is highly correlated with decreased levels of the reproductive hormone testosterone, both of which are typical causes of infertility.

Observe Your Digestive Wellness.

More than 100 trillion friendly bacteria live in your stomach, and they create a wide range of metabolites that can have both beneficial and bad effects on hormone health. Your gut microbiota controls insulin resistance and sensations of fullness to regulate hormones.

For instance, your gut microbiota creates short-chain fatty acids (SCFAs) like butyrate, propionate, and acetate when it ferments fiber. Because they increase the burning of calories, acetate, and butyrate may help prevent insulin resistance and aid in weight management. By raising the hormones GLP-1 and PYY, which are associated with fullness, acetate, and butyrate may also control feelings of fullness.

Cut Back On The Sugar You Eat.

Reducing the amount of added sugar you eat may help you avoid obesity, diabetes, and other disorders while also maximizing hormone function. Several forms of sugar contain the simple sugar fructose, which is found in up to 43% of honey, 50% of refined table sugar, 55% of high fructose corn syrup, and 90% of agave.

Furthermore, the main sources of added sugars in the Western diet are beverages sweetened with sugar, and fructose is frequently utilized in soft drinks, fruit juice, and energy and sports drinks on a commercial basis.

Hormones & Diet in Women

Since about 1980, fructose intake has skyrocketed in the US, and research continuously demonstrates that consuming additional sugar increases insulin resistance, at least in part for reasons that are unrelated to overall calorie intake or weight gain. Prolonged use of fructose has been associated with changes in the gut microbiota, perhaps resulting in additional hormonal abnormalities.

Try Some Stress-Reduction Strategies.

Stress affects hormones in a number of ways. Because it helps your body deal with chronic stress, the hormone cortisol is also referred to as the stress hormone. Stress sets off a series of physiological reactions in your body that result in the generation of cortisol. The response usually ends when the stressor has subsided. However persistent stress degrades the feedback systems that assist in restoring the normalcy of your hormonal systems and are a reliable source. Consequently, prolonged stress keeps cortisol levels high.

A reliable source that boosts hunger and encourages you to eat more high-fat and sugary meals. Obesity and an excessive calorie intake may result from this. Furthermore, the synthesis of glucose from non-carbohydrate sources, or gluconeogenesis, is stimulated by high cortisol levels and may result in insulin resistance.

Take In Good Fats.

Your diet may benefit from including high-quality natural fats to help lower insulin resistance and appetite. Unlike other fats, medium-chain triglycerides (MCTs) are more likely to be absorbed by your liver for instant use as energy rather than being stored in adipose tissue, which increases calorie burning. Additionally, MCTs are less likely to encourage insulin resistance. Furthermore, by lowering inflammation and pro-inflammatory indicators, healthy fats like omega-3s can improve insulin sensitivity. Hence, research indicates that omega-3s may stop the rise in cortisol levels that occur during stress.

Pure MCT oil, avocados, almonds, peanuts, macadamia nuts, hazelnuts, fatty fish, and olive and coconut oils are good sources of these good fats.

Obtain Regular, Excellent Sleep

Getting adequate restful sleep is essential for overall health, regardless of how consistent your workout program is or how nourishing your food is. Hormone abnormalities, including those in insulin, cortisol, leptin, ghrelin, and HGH, have been related to inadequate sleep.

For example, getting too little sleep reduces insulin sensitivity, but it also raises cortisol levels over the course of a day, which might cause insulin resistance.

CHAPTER 6
Reproductive Hormone Mechanism

Estrogen is the female sex hormone that causes puberty and aids in menstrual cycle regulation, pregnancy maintenance, cholesterol control, and maintaining healthy bones. Testosterone is the male sex hormone that causes changes during puberty; it also boosts muscle strength, bone density, and sex drive in both sexes. Testosterone is produced by the ovaries and testicles. The levels of testosterone produced can have an impact on your physical and emotional well-being. A hormone called testosterone is present in both humans and other animals.

The primary source of testosterone in men is the testicles. In far smaller quantities, the ovaries of women also produce testosterone. During puberty, testosterone production starts to rise dramatically and then starts to decline around the age of thirty. Testosterone is essential for the development of sperm and is most commonly linked to sex drive.

Hormones & Diet in Women

It also has an impact on red blood cell formation, bone and muscle mass, and how men store fat in their bodies. A man's mood might also be influenced by his testosterone levels.

Low Amounts Of Testosterone

Men who have low testosterone, or low T levels, may have a range of symptoms, such as:

- A decline in sexual desire
- Reduced vigor
- Gaining mass
- Depressive sensations
- Sultriness
- Low sense of worth
- Reduced body hair
- less dense bones

Hormone levels might decline due to several circumstances, even if a man's natural production of testosterone naturally decreases with age. Testicular damage and cancer therapies like radiation or chemotherapy can have a detrimental effect on the synthesis of testosterone.

Long-term medical conditions and stress can also reduce the synthesis of testosterone. A few of these consist of:

- HIV
- kidney illness
- Alcohol Abuse
- Cilia in the liver

Testosterone In Mature Women,

In women, testosterone levels gradually decrease; nonetheless, low T levels can also result in a range of symptoms, such as:

• Low desire

• A decrease in bone density

• Inability to focus

• Despondency

Pituitary, hypothalamic, and adrenal gland disorders, as well as ovarian excision, can all result in low T levels in females.

Women with low T levels may be administered testosterone therapy; however, it is uncertain if this treatment is beneficial for enhancing postmenopausal women's sexual or cognitive functioning.

Tension And Mood

Cortisol: During stressful situations, cortisol is released, which raises heart rate and blood pressure. Excessive levels are harmful to your health and are commonly known as the "stress hormone."

Adrenaline: Stress triggers the release of this "fight or flight" hormone, which quickens heart rate.

Melatonin: This hormone helps the body get ready for sleep by being released at night. It is frequently referred to as our "sleep-inducing hormone."

CHAPTER 7
Best Foods That Balances Hormones

Cruciferous Veggies

"Eating cruciferous vegetables regularly can help prevent the development of estrogen-dominant cancers. Broccoli and broccoli sprouts are excellent at assisting our livers in metabolizing estrogen efficiently and healthily. Kale, cabbage, bok choy, cauliflower, and Brussels sprouts are more cruciferous vegetables. Try them in our broccoli-cauliflower soup or roast them with a sprinkle of olive oil, which helps boost the absorption of vitamins A, D, E, and K. Tuna and salmon albacore. Hormone building blocks are fat and cholesterol. To produce the sex hormones testosterone and estrogen, you must have adequate cholesterol. Selecting lipids rich in omega-3s and minimizing saturated fats are crucial, as is eliminating trans fats. Omega-3 fatty acids can be found in abundance in salmon, tinned albacore tuna, walnuts, flaxseed, olive oil, avocados, and chia seeds.

"In addition to balancing your appetite hormones, salmon also helps control female testosterone levels since it contains a lot of vitamin D. Fish's healthy fats enhance the body's overall hormonal communication. Hormones are the means by which the endocrine system communicates with the brain, improving our mood and cognitive abilities.

Guacamole

"Avocados are loaded with beta-sitosterol, which can positively affect blood cholesterol levels and help balance cortisol," Gabriel explains. According to a 2019 study, the fat and fiber in avocados raised levels of satiety-promoting hormones such as cholecystokinin (CCK), peptide YY (PYY), and glucagon-like peptide 1 (GLP-1). "The plant sterols in avocados also influence estrogen and progesterone, the two hormones responsible for regulating ovulation and menstrual cycles." Add half an avocado to your breakfast or lunch to make you feel full for hours. These healthy avocado recipes also call for avocado.

Hormones & Diet in Women

Fruits and vegetables, preferably organic.

"According to studies, fertility is harmed by even one serving of a fruit or vegetable heavy in pesticides, like strawberries. Many pesticides act as hormone disruptors, meaning they either mimic hormones in your body or they affect the actions of your hormones."

Glyphosate, for example, has a long history of being shown to be an endocrine disruptor. It is crucial to stay away from endocrine-disrupting chemicals, and eating organic food can significantly lower your exposure to them. Consider shopping organic on the Environmental Working Group's "Dirty Dozen" list, which ranks the most contaminated produce.

Minimize exposure if possible, but know that all fruits and vegetables are rich in vitamins, minerals, and antioxidants.

It is noteworthy to note that the benefits of eating fruits and vegetables far outweigh not eating them if you can't afford to eat organic.

High-Fiber Sweet Potatoes

Consider whole grains, fruits, and vegetables. "A diet rich in fiber can aid in the removal of excess hormones from the body." "At most meals, aim to include half of your plate with nonstarchy veggies and a quarter with starchy vegetables, such as whole grains or potatoes. Whole grains and legumes, as well as root vegetables like carrots, sweet potatoes, and squash, can be beneficial." Smith adds that consuming some grain with dinner may aid in the regulation of the hormones cortisol and melatonin. "Some carbs can help mitigate elevated cortisol levels.

Bacteria And Probiotics

The gut is the body's largest endocrine organ, producing and secreting over 20 hormones related to hunger, satiety, and metabolism. Prebiotics are the good bacteria that live in the gut, and probiotics are the fibrous foods those bacteria eat to grow.

Smith suggests eating prebiotic foods like raw garlic and oats, asparagus, dandelion, almonds, apples, bananas, Jerusalem artichokes, and chicory, as well as probiotics like kimchi and yogurt.

Foods that are bad for hormone balance

"Research reveals that downing artificial sweeteners may modify our gut bacteria, which may impact the balance of appetite and fullness, the same chemicals as leptin and ghrelin. This means that eating fewer processed meals, fried foods, sugar, and artificial sweeteners and drinking less alcohol will help prevent hormone imbalances.

Alcohol disrupts several hormonal functions, including the metabolism of estrogen and blood sugar regulation. Alcohol consumption is linked to a higher chance of developing breast cancer, in addition to other malignancies.

Limit your intake to no more than one drink for women and two for men each day, respectively. Exercise, sleep, and stress.

Hormones & Diet in Women

Hormone balance also depends on maintaining a good diet, getting enough sleep, reducing stress, and engaging in regular exercise. Lack of sleep interferes with leptin and ghrelin, which is why you tend to seek carbohydrates and all foods when you're weary. It has also been related to reduced testosterone in men. Prolonged stress raises cortisol levels, which can induce hypertension and inhibit the immunological and digestive systems. Carb cravings are also caused by cortisol. Increased norepinephrine and serotonin levels are caused by exercise, meditation, and sleep, and we like that suggestion of eating chocolate. Serotonin is the "feel-good" hormone, and norepinephrine gives you more energy.

CHAPTER 8
Hormonal Imbalances' Fundamental Causes

The following are the core reasons for these imbalances that the two doctors discussed in a recent podcast with Dr. Mark Hyman:

Toxic stress: They emphasize how toxic stress can result in either high or low cortisol levels and can cause hypo- or hyperactivity (i.e., an underactive or hyperactive thyroid).

Reproductive Years: Estrogen and progesterone levels may drop during the postpartum and perimenopause periods. A high-sugar, starchy diet can lead to insulin resistance, which can result in the belly weight gain that so many women struggle to lose.

Endocrine disruptors: Plastics, pesticides, and herbicides contain environmental chemicals that can cause endocrine disruption. Dairy hormones have also been connected to a problem.

Hormones & Diet in Women

The appropriate functioning of our hormones is adversely affected by all these circumstances.

Resolving Women's Hormonal Imbalances

For women's hormones, a ketogenic diet that includes carbohydrates from nutrient-dense foods like cruciferous vegetables is advised. Since fat is the primary component of sex hormones, many women also do not consume enough fat in their diets. Women are to follow a diet consisting of 60–70% fat, less than 25 grams of net carbs, and 20% protein for four weeks. This diet should not cause feelings of hunger or deprivation because fat slows down the emptying of the stomach, which increases feelings of fullness. Even though 25 grams of net carbohydrates a day is not much, obtaining these carbohydrates, especially from high-fiber, cruciferous vegetables will satisfy your hunger and meet your nutritional demands.

CHAPTER 9
Hormones and Ketosis

With the help of this diet, your body can go into ketosis and start using fat for energy instead of glucose. In addition to supporting the health of hormones, nutritional ketosis reduces inflammation, promotes weight reduction, improves energy, and improves mental clarity and sleep. Researchers have acknowledged that women might find it difficult to maintain this diet over time and that it is not appropriate for everyone. But if you give it a go for four weeks, you'll be able to experience metabolic flexibility, which means your body may alternate between burning fat and glucose for energy depending on what you're consuming and the fuel available.

Building Strength as We Get Older

Strength exercise is strongly advised in addition to diet to help women maintain and gain muscle mass as they age.

Researchers suggest doing one-third of your weekly workout as cardio and two-thirds as strength training. Not to be disregarded, muscle mass is one of the most significant indicators of general health.

CHAPTER 10
Intercity Fasting: A Safe Method for Detoxing and Healthy Eating

There are many detoxification, cleansing, and fasting programs available. Wellness celebrities promote intricate deprivation exercises. However, under the pretense of self-care, fruit and vegetable juice-based daylong fasts might promote disordered eating. Furthermore, fresh juices lack the protein, fat, and fiber necessary to maintain normal bodily functions, despite their high vitamin and mineral content. However, an increasing amount of evidence suggests that eating fresh, complete meals isn't the only thing that contributes to metabolic health.

Based on circadian rhythms, one type of daily fasting may help your digestive system get off to a faster start. Eating a diet changes your metabolism a bit of a misnomer, intermittent fasting conjures up images of missing lunches and lemon water.

However, in intermittent fasting, "fast" refers to a healthy time each day when you don't eat that is, after supper, before breakfast, and while you sleep. Put another way, studies on intermittent fasting, or more precisely, circadian rhythm eating, indicate that irregular meals, late-night nibbling, and all-day grazing are detrimental to human health.

This is because, like all bodily systems, our digestive system (as well as the microorganisms it harbors) runs on a 24-hour cycle and needs rest intervals to stay healthy. Consuming food during these intervals of rest that are programmable by genetics strains the pancreas, which secretes insulin, which transfers sugar from the bloodstream to the cells.

Any remaining sugar is subsequently stored by insulin in your muscles and liver. You gain weight if your liver turns the excess sugar that it receives into fat. While decreased insulin levels caused by fasting aid in fat burning, persistently rising insulin levels caused by all-day snacking are associated with an increased risk of cardiovascular disease in adolescents and young adults.

Fasting periods also reduce blood pressure, promote cellular repair that wards off infection, deterioration, and malignant growth, and raise growth hormone levels, which contribute to the creation of muscle.

Chapter 11
How to Exactly Detox Your Body for Hormone Balancing Naturally
How to cleanse the body and control hormones

You can aid your body in producing more natural hormones and enhance detoxification to help restore hormone balance. This six-step process provides a starting point for treating all aspects of your health that are often associated with insufficient hormone function, however, there are various ways to go about it.

Step 1: Go For Daily Strolls

Studies have shown that exercise helps regulate a number of hormones, including insulin, cortisol, thyroid hormones, and others. Exercise not only improves hormone-affecting pollutant detoxification but also promotes sweating.

How to commence: Establish a routine that pushes you without becoming too strenuous. Never forget to give yourself days off. Chronic inflammation can be brought on by excessive exercise coupled with inadequate sleep, and this can then impact hormone production and imbalance.

Step 2: Lower Your Tension

For your body, stress is the ultimate junk food. You can follow all the "right" procedures and eat the healthiest food, but hormone problems can still arise if you give your body a daily dose of stress.

Your body's primary stress hormone, cortisol, rises when you are under stress as a normal, healthy reaction to shield you from the trying circumstances. The issue arises from the fact that while you are under constant stress, your body is unable to revert to its natural condition of tranquility. Adrenal exhaustion, poor metabolic health, and other hormone issues including insulin resistance might result from these persistently elevated cortisol levels.

What you can do: Everyone encounters stressful circumstances occasionally. Introduce stress-relieving practices such as breathwork and meditation (there are some excellent applications like Headspace and Calm that you can use anytime, anywhere). Afterwards, what? Consider what is causing you the most stress and try to find solutions to rearrange your schedule.

Perhaps now is the right moment to give those toxic people in your life some limits!

Step 3. Get More Slumber

Hormone balance depends on sleep. In fact, it has been demonstrated (1) that insufficient sleep directly contributes to hormone abnormalities. Which is worse still? Inadequate sleep can also be prolonged by hormonal abnormalities. We need to make getting the suggested 7 hours of sleep every night a priority if we want to break free from this vicious cycle.

But it might be difficult when there are a lot of things that can make it difficult for you to achieve restful, uninterrupted sleep.

Your body produces less melatonin in the evening, which is a "sleepy time" hormone that helps you wind down, and more cortisol in the middle of the night, which keeps you wide awake. These factors include light pollution and blue light exposure.

Hormones & Diet in Women

What you can do: With increased studies being conducted on the benefits of sleep, a plethora of innovative products aimed at improving the quality and duration of sleep are now available. Products such as blue-light-blocking spectacles and blackout curtains can assist in minimizing light pollution and allow technology use prior to bedtime without influencing melatonin levels.

Step 4: Examine Your Food

For the creation of hormones, your body needs a particular ratio of macro and micronutrients. I frequently discover that dietary inadequacies are the cause of many people's hormone abnormalities in my telehealth functional medicine clinic.

As an illustration, vitamin D deficiency is one of the most widespread nutritional deficits worldwide, despite being one of the primary elements required for healthy hormone production! I also see how the myth that "fat is bad" will play out in the long run.

While America continues to struggle to move past the outdated notion that picking low-fat foods is the healthiest choice, healthy fats are necessary for the creation of hormones.

What you can do: is increase your intake of whole foods, avocados, walnuts, and coconut oil; you can also increase your intake of foods high in vitamin D, such as eggs and wild-caught salmon. Supplements like D3-K2 and Omega+ might be useful when taken in conjunction with dietary adjustments to overcome deficiencies because sometimes you just need a little additional help.

Step 5: Consider Using Vitamins

Hormone imbalances are typically treated in conventional medicine with drugs like birth control. Regretfully, these have no effect on the underlying cause of your hormone imbalances rather, they merely serve as a band-aid solution.

Hormones & Diet in Women

Functional medicine focuses on treatments like clinically supported natural supplements that have been demonstrated to restore hormone balance, rather than adding more drugs that come with their own set of adverse effects. There are supplements available that have been researched for their potential to help with fatigue and female hormone imbalances like estrogen dominance. The best thing you can do is look into adaptogens. The majority of people can safely use these plant and herbal remedies, which are well-known for their ability to balance hormones and reduce stress. There are numerous types of adaptogens that support various aspects of your health, so you're sure to discover one that works for the symptoms you're experiencing. If you are pregnant or nursing, make sure to consult your physician before starting any new medications.

Step 6: Remove Poisons

Eliminating pollutants as much as you can is my top recommendation for supporting your hormones.

Hormones & Diet in Women

Our environment is getting more and more poisonous, and this bombardment of toxins has been connected to serious hormone issues. For instance, plastic, cosmetics, and cleaning items for the home all contain xenoestrogens. Your body produces more estrogen as a result of these artificial compounds acting as estrogen, which also makes it more difficult for your body to properly break down and get rid of extra estrogen. The thousands of additional substances that can cause hormone abnormalities, such as pesticides, PCBs, plastics, heavy metals, and more, are not even considered in this.

What you can do: is purge yourself of everything. Although it is impossible to completely eliminate toxins, you can lessen their effects by doing everything in your power to assist your body's natural detoxification processes.

The Benefits Of Functional Medicine

There is no "one-size-fits-all" method to healing, despite the fact that I say this a lot. particularly in regard to hormone abnormalities. Rebalancing hormones can be achieved in a number of ways, but the best approach is to support your unique detoxification process. We perform a variety of hormone lab tests in my telemedicine functional medicine clinic to provide a clear picture of the underlying issues. We can tailor recommendations to target the areas of your life that require support by identifying the cause of your hormone abnormalities. We view hormone health through the prism of bio-individuality, regardless of the cause poor sleep or dietary modifications, for example.

CHAPTER 12
Ways To Reduce Weight Without Becoming Starvy

If you experience intense cravings, have digestive issues like heartburn or frequent bloating, get angry when you're hungry (also known as "hangry"), feel like your metabolism has slowed down with age, or have trouble falling or staying asleep, it may be worth a try to implement the circadian diet. Go slowly if you choose to give it a try. The majority of people fast for 12–9 hours and eat during a window of 12–15 hours. To give your digestive organs time to heal, the circadian diet suggests cutting your eating window down to 8–10 hours and eating genuine meals spaced out by breaks. Starting with a 12-hour eating window and reducing it by an hour each day until you're at eight, or nine, or 10 if eight feels too restrictive, is a major change.

After thirty days, evaluate your feelings. Good? Then you are welcome to proceed. Poor? Modify your eating routine until you start to feel better. Eating a nutritious and filling amount of food every day is one of the best things about circadian eating. Instead of a yo-yo diet, it's a shift in lifestyle.

CHAPTER 13
Short-Term Circadian Diet: Eat A Heavier Breakfast

So, to follow a circadian diet, how do you plan your meals? Especially for those of us who work 9 to 5 jobs (who wants to eat supper at work?), it's not simple.

Try making breakfast your largest meal of the day and think about bringing it to work (along with lunch), as studies have shown that our bodies are better at controlling blood sugar, digesting, and burning calories in the morning. In this manner, you'll have plenty of time to prepare dinner at home and be able to extend your dining window. Rich in fiber and packed with nutrients, healthy fats like avocado and full-fat yogurt pair well with high-fiber grains like brown rice to keep you feeling full for longer.

You can extend your feeling of fullness until lunch by adding an egg, some tofu, and some fruit.

This calorie-dense green smoothie recipe is a great option if you feel awkward having breakfast at your desk.

Dietary Circadian Smoothie

- One handful of young spinach
- Two oranges
- Half a cup of almond milk
- Two times
- Three tablespoons of almond or peanut butter
- 1/4 cup plain yogurt with added fat
- One eighth teaspoon cinnamon
- One dash of salt
- Taste and adjust the ratios, then combine and serve immediately.

Reduce your calorie intake and portion sizes at lunch, and for optimal effects, have a light meal once you get home.

Try to consume only fruits, vegetables, whole grains, lean protein, and healthy fats such as those found in nuts, seeds, olive oil, or fatty fish throughout the day.

Herbs for Optimal Metal Success. Several herbs might help your body's natural metabolism. According to a 2018 study, matcha green tea's caffeine and catechin content can speed up fat burning when exercising.

Additionally, green tea may help control blood sugar, preventing mood swings and appetite surges. Seek out expertly mixed blends that include extra herbs such as liquorice root and dandelion in addition to green tea. Studies on animals suggest that dandelion may lower blood levels of sugar and fat, while a review of 26 clinical trials indicated that liquorice ingestion lowers body mass index (BMI).

Circadian Rhythm Diet: Advantages And Disadvantages

The goal of the circadian diet is to purposefully and reliably satiate your appetite. Beyond the health advantages, maintaining daily meals and rest periods respects rather than undermines the therapeutic properties of food. Having said that, not everyone is a good fit for the circadian diet. Avoid it if you are pregnant, above the age of 70, brittlely diabetic, under the age of 21, have a low Body Mass Index (BMI), have a history of eating disorders, or have kidney or cardiac issues.

Hormones & Diet in Women

If your daily energy levels, appetite patterns, digestion, and sleep are all within an acceptable range, we also suggest the "aren't broke, don't fix it approach". Although the science underlying the circadian diet is fascinating, each person is unique, so if you already feel well, you probably do.

SUMMARY

Hormones affect many aspects of life, including mood, energy, hunger, weight, growth and development, metabolism, digestion, and reproduction. Hormone balance is maintained by eating a diet rich in fruits, vegetables, whole grains, healthy fats, and protein. Hormone disruption can result from eating too few calories overall, fiber, healthy fats, or healthy fats. This can cause obesity, diabetes, infertility, and cancer. Alcohol, stress, sleep deprivation, and processed meals can also affect the gut microbiota, which regulates hormone balance, and cause direct or indirect hormonal disruption. Women no longer have to accept aging as a passive process; instead, they may take charge of their health and well-being and live stronger, healthier, more empowered lives.